Sleep, Baby, Sleep

The Six Bs for a Great Sleeping Baby

Veronica L. Esposito

ISBN 979-8-88851-233-3 (Paperback)
ISBN 979-8-88851-235-7 (Hardcover)
ISBN 979-8-88851-234-0 (Digital)

First Edition

Covenant Books
11661 Hwy 707
Murrells Inlet, SC 29576
www.covenantbooks.com

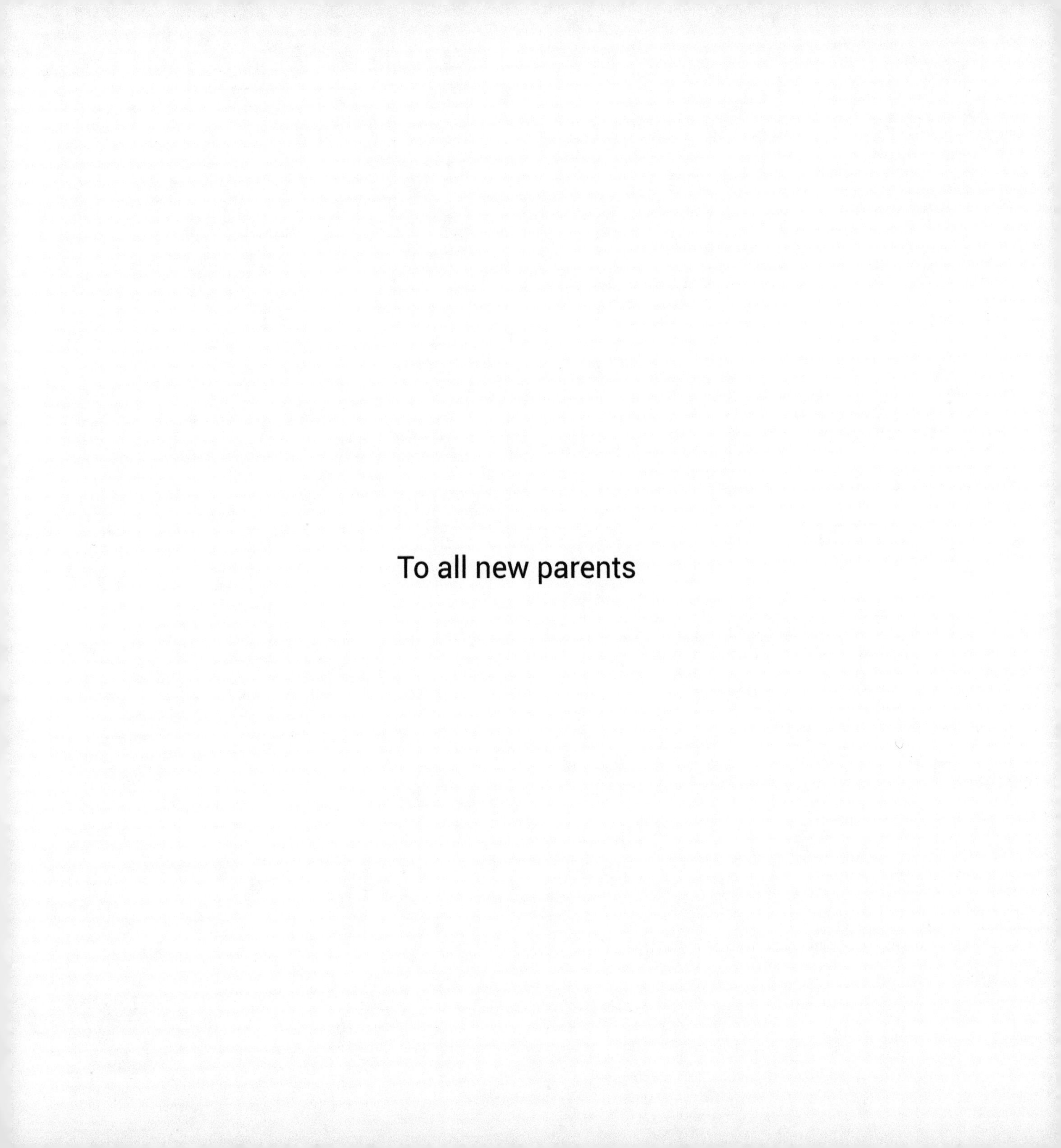
To all new parents

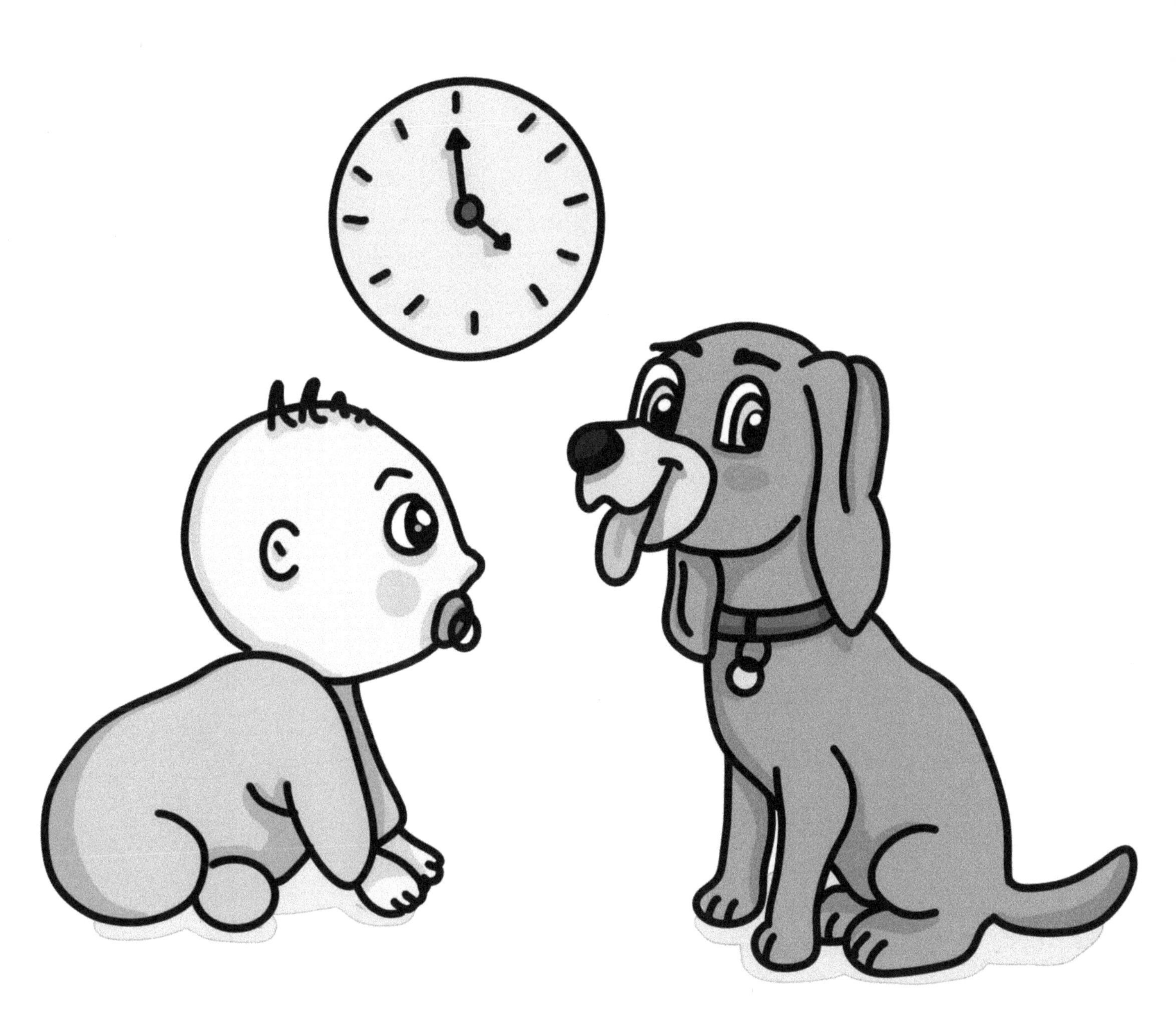

Babies, like puppies, cannot tell the time, but these nightly steps will work for you fine.

Breast or Bottle

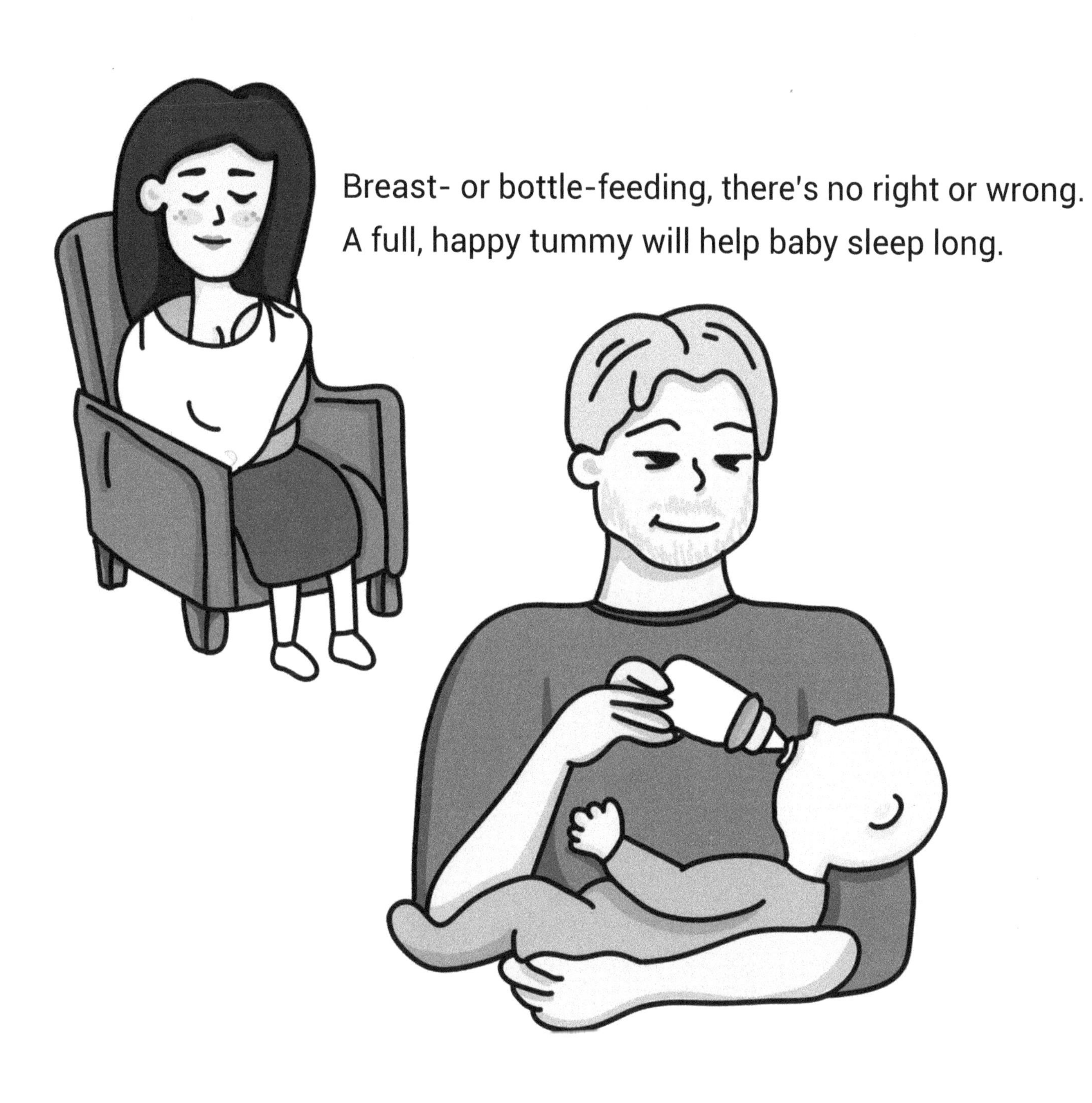

Breast- or bottle-feeding, there's no right or wrong.
A full, happy tummy will help baby sleep long.

Bath Time

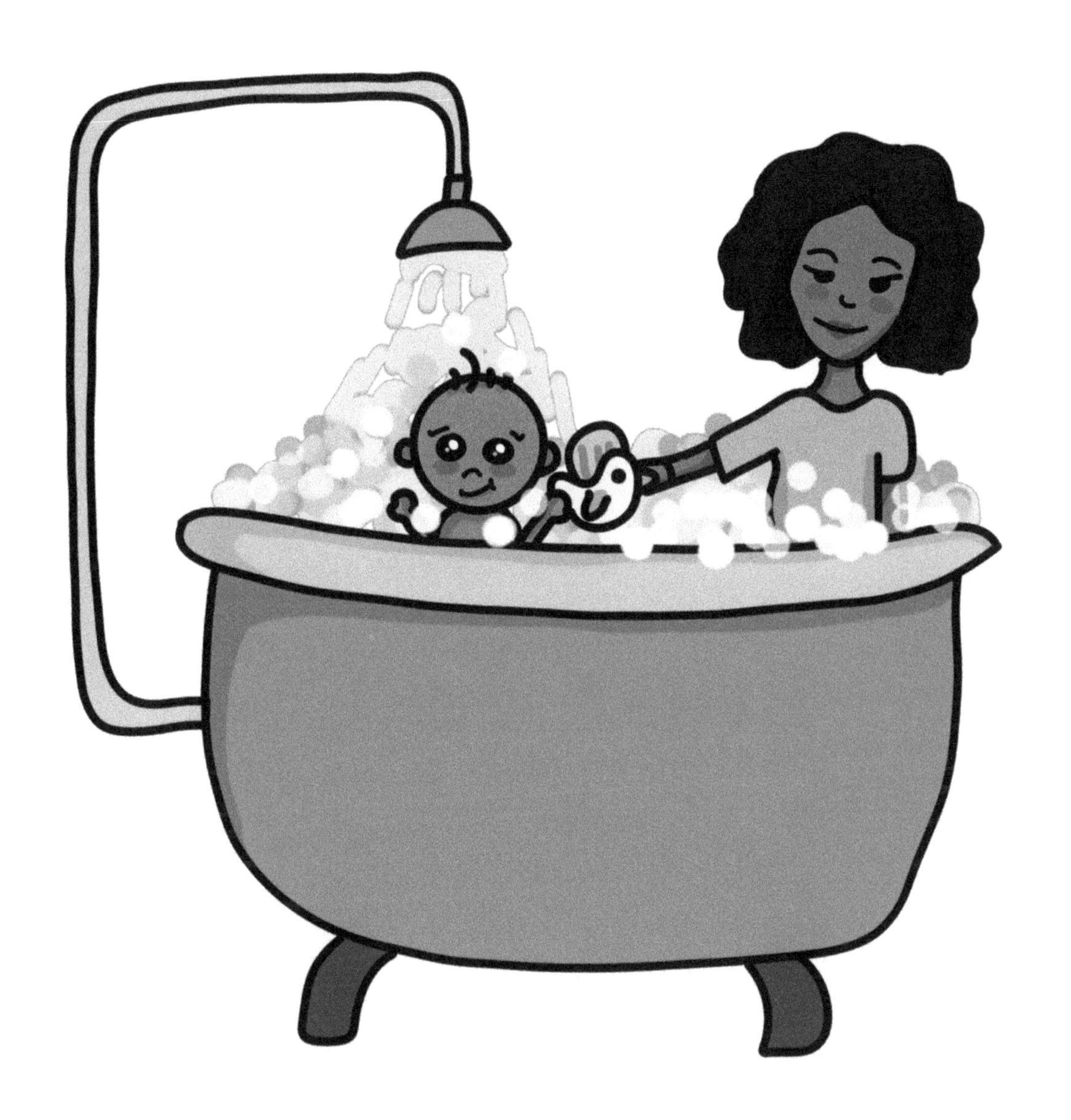

Water and bubbles, bath time is fun.
Daily, at first, is how it is done.

Brush Teeth

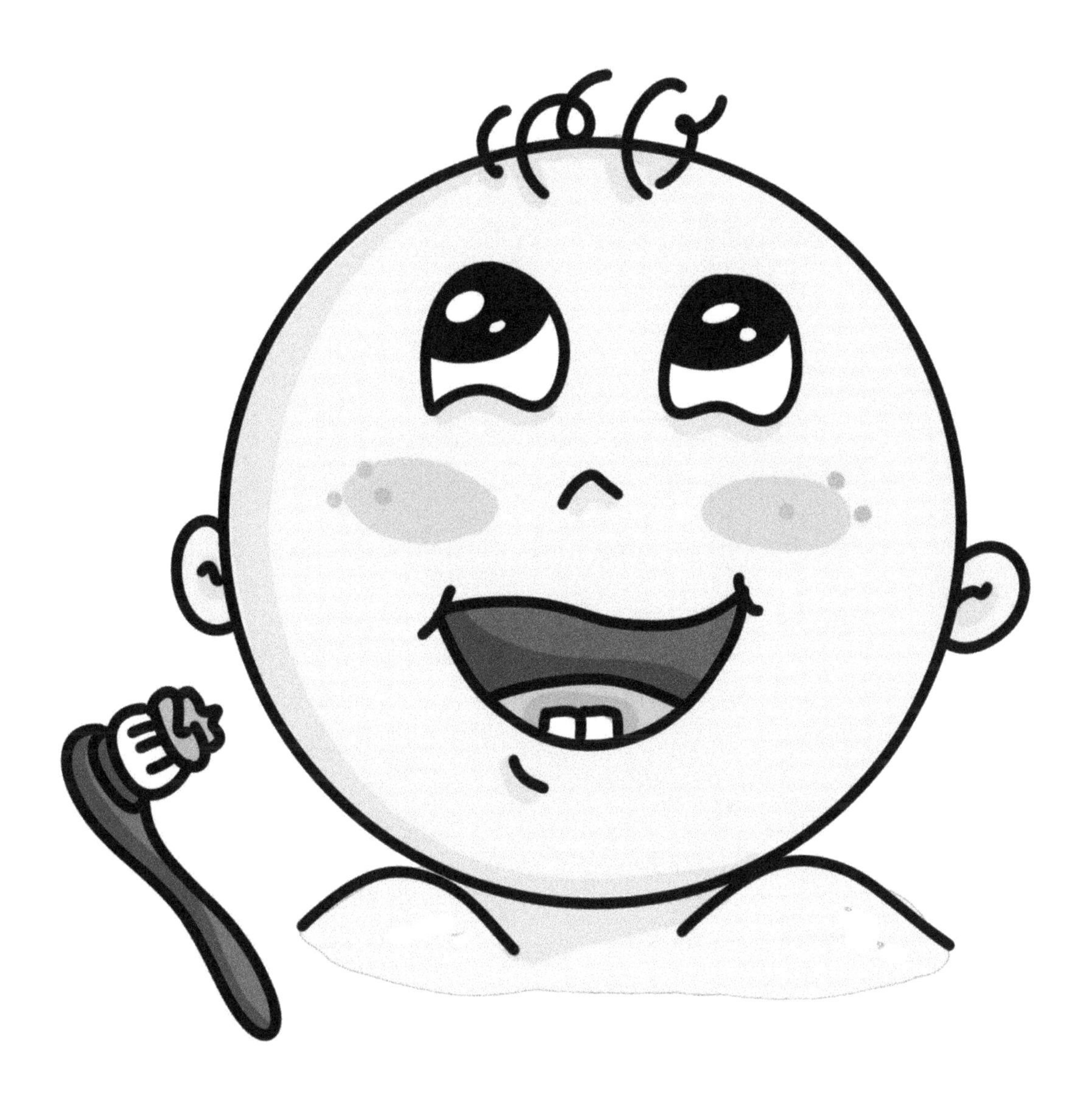

Brushing their teeth is certainly key,
To having great brushers at one, two, and three.

Book

Bedtime reading helps baby unwind,
And will foster the love of reading each time.

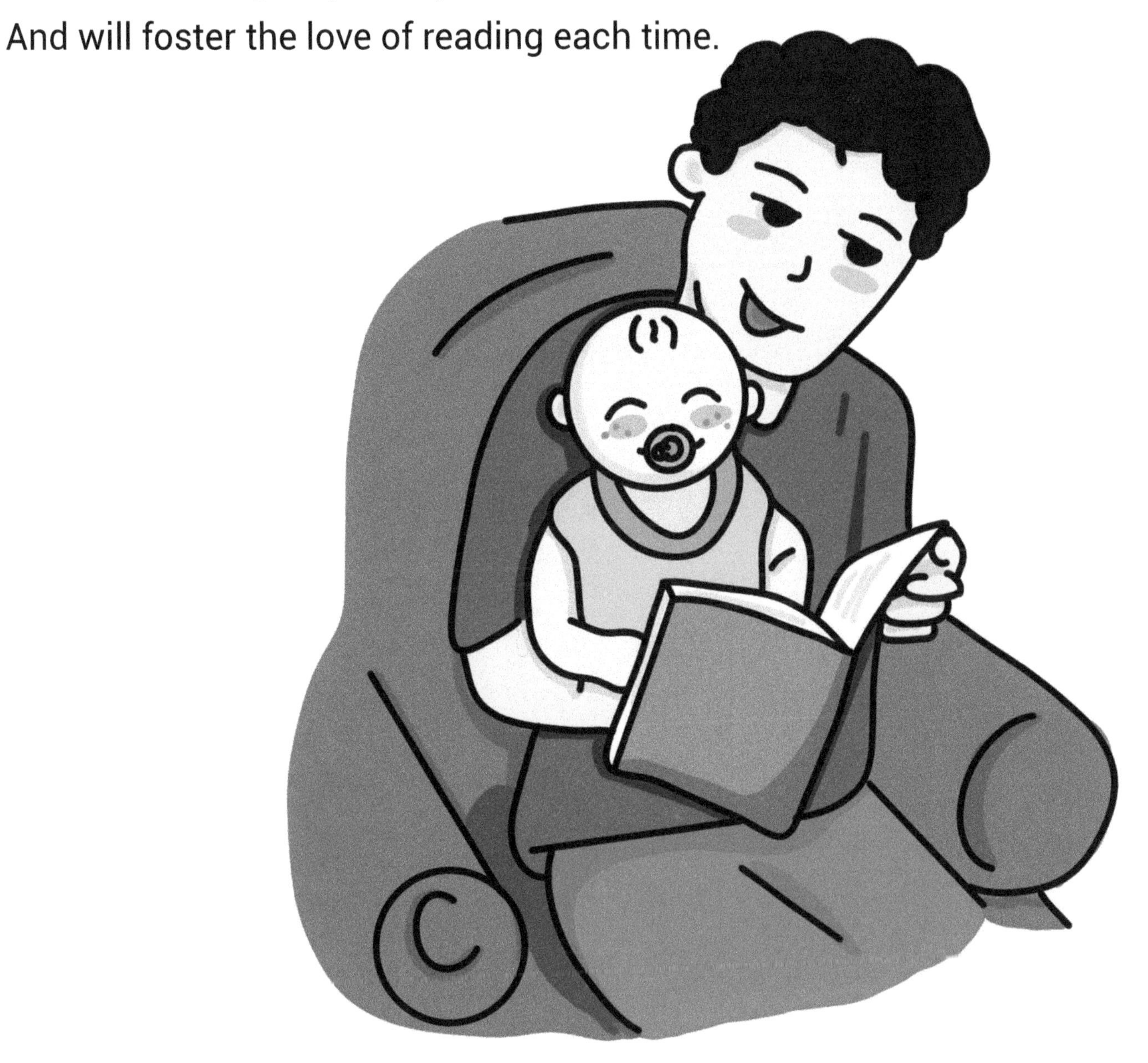

Blessings

Counting your blessings is a definite must,
Being grateful to God and learning to trust.

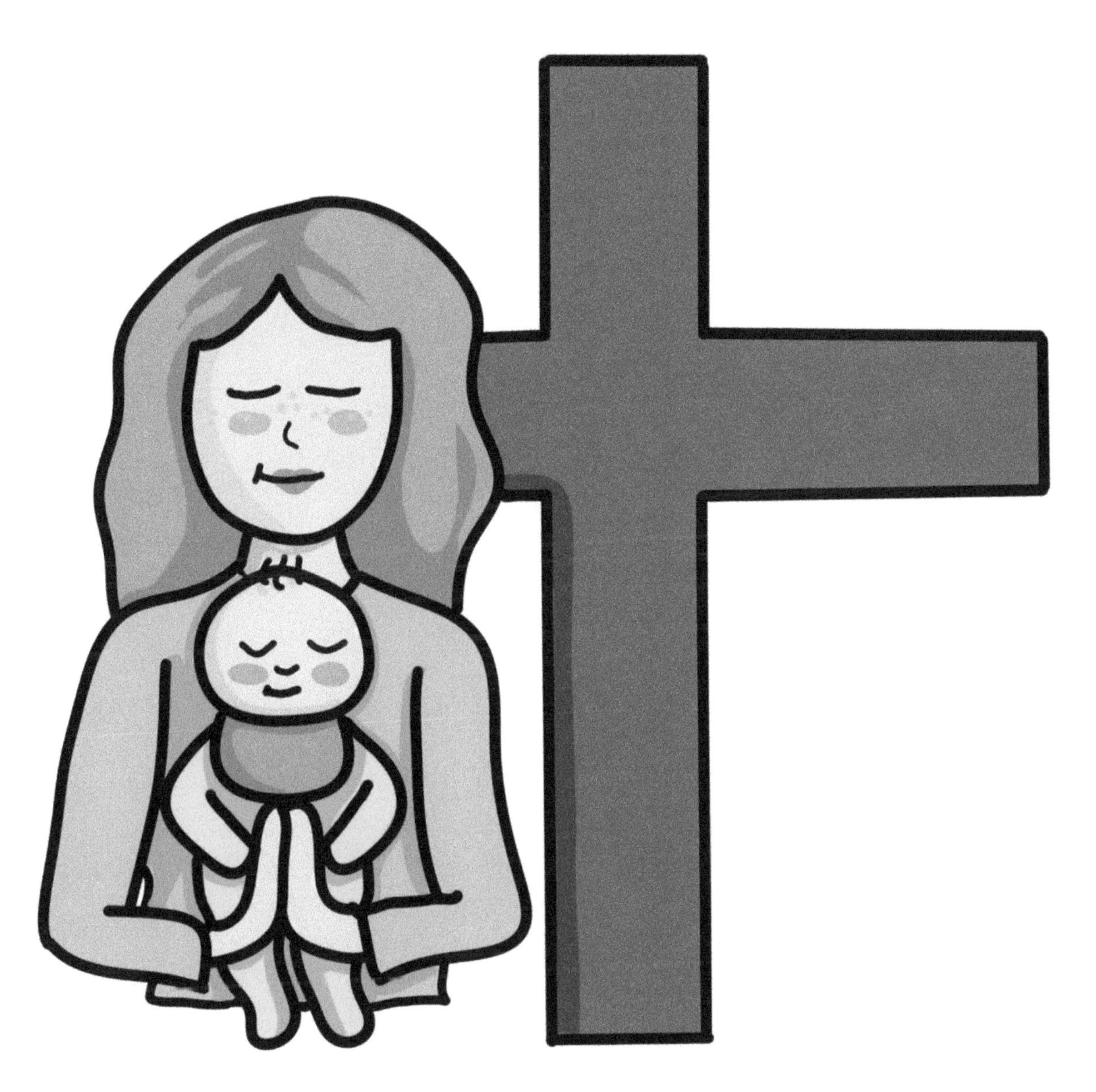

Bed

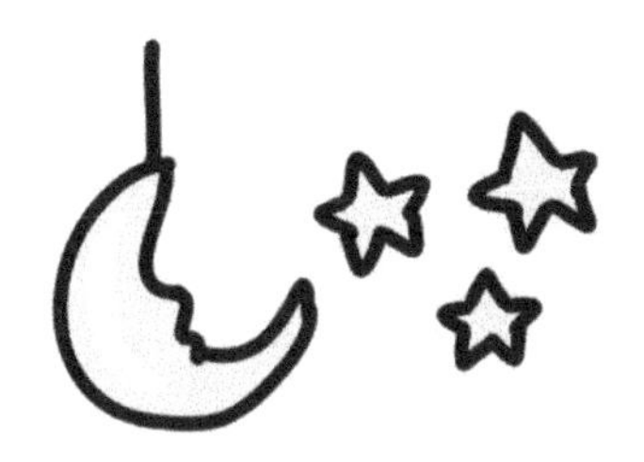

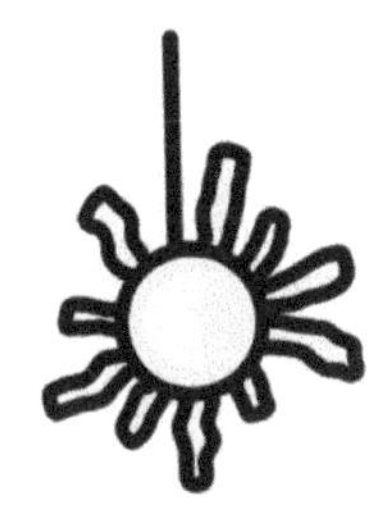

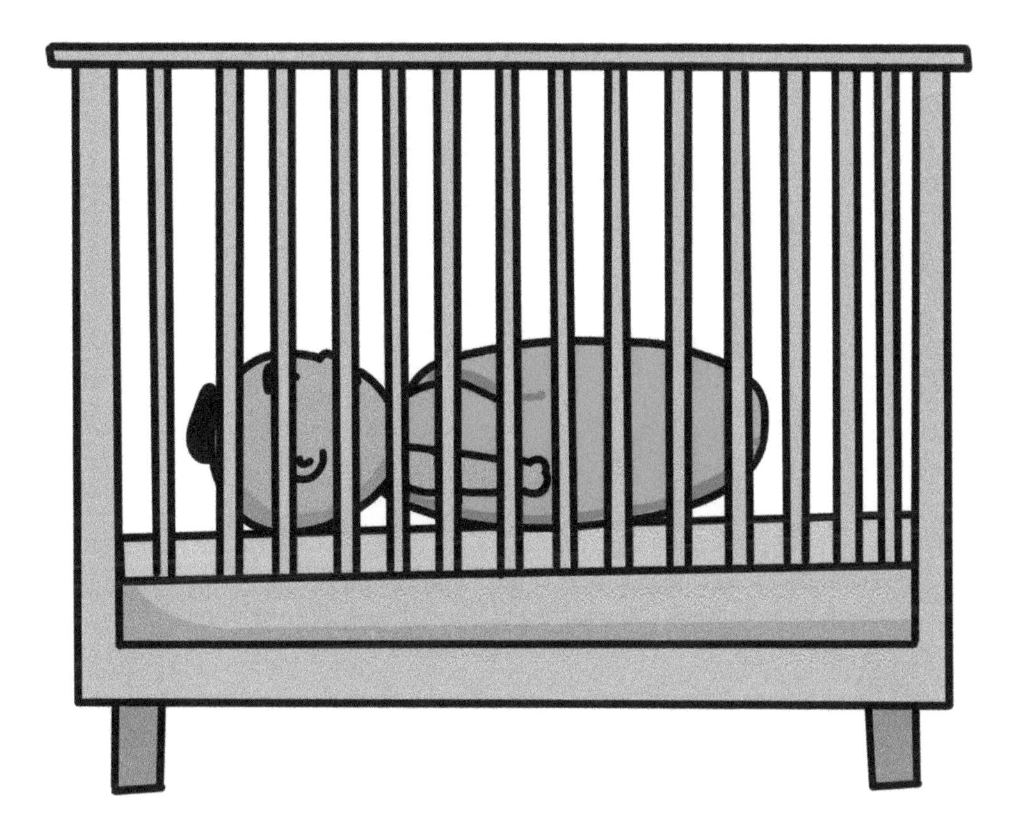

Now, it is time to place them alone in their bed.

Sleep, baby, sleep,

Rest your sweet head.

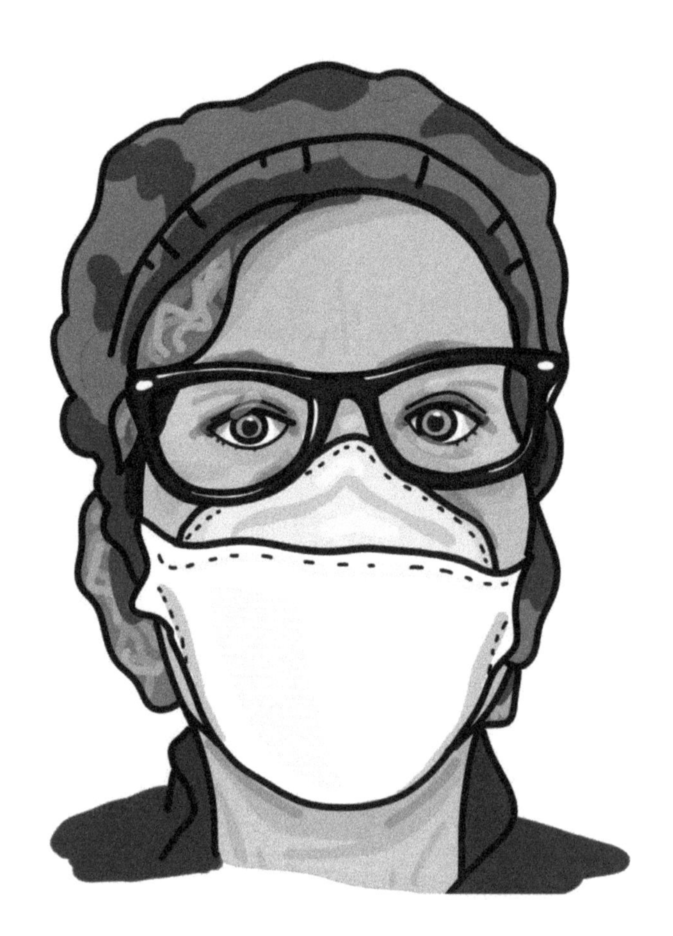

Hi, my name is Ronnie.
A certified pediatric registered nurse and
mom for thirty-two-plus years.
These six daily steps,
Tested, tried, and true.
A well-rested baby,
Makes a happier you.

Acknowledgments

I'd like to thank God for the gift of my loving, supportive husband, Frank, our family, and my amazing career as a nurse. Creating our recipe together as parents—a lifetime of love, support, and tireless nights with our sons, Matt and Nick.

Lastly, I'd like to thank my godchild and niece, Rachel. Without her guidance, this would not have been possible.

About the Author

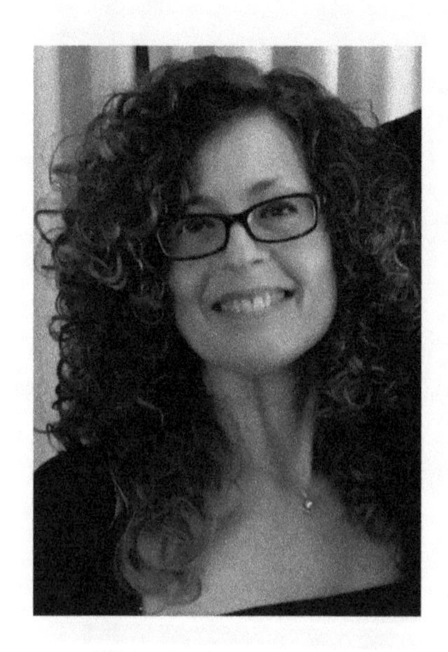

Veronica Lynne Esposito, or Nurse Ronnie, as her patients and their families would call her, is an experienced mother of two grown sons and a seasoned maternal child-health / certified pediatric registered nurse for over thirty-two years. She is well versed in the areas of both the mothering and patient care of the newborn, infant, toddler, and child.

In 2015, she was humbly awarded the Johanna McCarthy Nursing Award, which recognizes those who exhibit excellence in nursing and high-quality patient care. This prestigious award was nominated to her by her colleagues for providing exemplary care to the pediatric population. Her colleague's choice words: "There is no doubt that Ronnie's years as a pediatric/maternal child nurse have provided her with the necessary skills to serve as an advocate for her patients and their families. She never fails to go the extra mile to facilitate a parent's hospital stay and consistently demonstrates compassion, empathy, devotion, and enthusiasm. The consummate team player, she never hesitates to lend a hand and provide advice for any problematic situation. She is very flexible, approachable, and knowledgeable. She has the gift of soothing both nervous parents as well as supporting physicians and colleagues under stressful circumstances."

Veronica Lynne and her husband live in the Hudson Valley, a suburb of New York. They have two grown children and one gentle giant, Sir Oswald of Netherwood. She loves spending time with her family, baking, gardening, and visiting her four-legged furry neighbors.